101 Bodyweight Workouts

Get Toned At Home Without Any Equipment

By Dominique & Erik Myers

SOCIAL MEDIA

Instagram

@mauifitcouple

TikTok

@mauifitcouple

GET IN TOUCH

domanderik4@gmail.com

Created by Dominique & Erik Myers

ISBN 9798639327049

Before you start this exercise program or make any changes in your lifestyle you must get your doctor or physician's approval. This product is for informational purposes only and is not meant as medical advice, nor is it a substitute for medical advice. In no way will Dominique or Erik Myers be held responsible for any injuries or problems that may occur due to the use of this program or advice contained within. Consult with a doctor before starting any exercise program. Performing exercise of all types can pose a risk to the exerciser. Before exercising make certain that the equipment is in good condition and be sure to know your own physical limits. Adequate warm up and cool downs should be undertaken before and after any exercise. If you experience any pain, discomfort, dizziness or shortness of breath, stop exercising immediately and consult your doctor. Please understand that you are solely responsible for the way information from 101 Body Weight Workouts by Dominique and Erik Myers is perceived and ultized and you do so at your own risk.

Your journey begins NOW.

These workouts were designed to make you sweat and push you to your limits.

Some of the most common excuses we hear from people who want to live a healthier life (but don't follow through) is that they don't have enough time, they don't have enough equipment, and/or they can't afford a gym membership...

With these 101 workouts, those excuses become irrelevant.

All the workouts can be done in 30 minutes or less, you don't need any equipment, and since you've already bought the book you're aware that we priced it fairly and affordably for everyone.

How you approach these workouts is entirely up to you. You can follow them in sequence from start to finish or pick and choose to your liking. You can do them at home or head to the gym and add some weights. You have the flexibility and freedom to fit these challenging workouts into your lifestyle accordingly.

Over the years our clients have made phenomenal progress with the workouts that you now possess and the reason why we made this book was for you to experience similar success.

Here are a few things to keep in mind as you begin:

• These workouts are designed to be completed at YOUR pace. Take rest breaks when needed and always be safe.

- Modify and adjust the exercises according to your skill set.

- If you'd like to increase the difficulty, feel free to add some weights or bands.

- If you're unfamiliar with a move, YouTube or Google it!

- You don't have to go through these workouts alone, invite friends and/or family members to complete them with you.

- If you feel like sharing your journey on social media, tag @mauifitcouple on Instagram so we can find your posts and cheer you on.

- If you'd like to be part of our (free) Fit Fam group on Facebook for support, accountability, and resources, we would love to have you. Request to join here: www.facebook.com/groups/mfcfitfam

- Once you finish all 101 workouts we invite you to do another round of them, try another one of our challenges, or email us (domanderik4@gmail.com) for a personalized program on our app.

- Have fun and stay safe!

Good luck and stay strong!
Dominique & Erik Myers

Workout #1

1st Set: 1 Round (Warm Up)
- ☐ 60 sec: Arm Circles
- ☐ 60 sec: Calf Raises

2nd Set: 2 Rounds
- ☐ 50 sec: Burpees
- ☐ 50 sec: Low Plank Alternating Side Punches
- ☐ 15 sec: Rest

3rd Set: 3 Rounds
- ☐ 40 sec: Thigh Slap Jumps
- ☐ 40 sec: Plank Toe Taps
- ☐ 15 sec: Rest

4th Set: 4 Rounds
- ☐ 30 sec: Jumping Lunges
- ☐ 30 sec: Diamond Push Ups
- ☐ 15 sec: Rest

5th Set: 5 Rounds
- ☐ 25 sec: Back & Forth Low Plank
- ☐ 25 sec: Knee Up Crunches
- ☐ 15 sec: Rest

6th Set: 6 Rounds
- ☐ 20 sec: Slow Push Ups
- ☐ 20 sec: High Plank
- ☐ 15 sec: Rest

7th Set: 7 Rounds
- ☐ 20 sec: Frog Burpees
- ☐ 10 sec: Rest

Workout #2

1st Set: 3 Rounds (Warm Up)
- ☐ 10 Push Ups
- ☐ 10 Squats
- ☐ 10 Crunches

2nd Set: 1 Round
- ☐ 100: Reverse Lunges (50 each side)
- ☐ 90: Shoulder Taps (45 each side)
- ☐ 80: High Knees (40 each side)
- ☐ 70: Calf Raises
- ☐ 60: Uppercut Punches (30 each side)
- ☐ 50: Shoelace Crunches
- ☐ 40: Prisoner Squats
- ☐ 30: Wide Push Ups
- ☐ 20: Bench Dips
- ☐ 10: Burpee Tuck Jumps

Workout #3

1st Set: 2 Rounds (Warm Up)
- ☐ 30 sec: High Knees
- ☐ 30 sec: Butt Kicks
- ☐ 10 sec: Rest

2nd Set: 3 Rounds
- ☐ 50 sec: Alternating Curtsy Lunges
- ☐ 10 sec: Rest
- ☐ 50 sec: Plank Pull Throughs
- ☐ 10 sec: Rest
- ☐ 30 sec: Burpee with Plank Jack

3rd Set: 3 Rounds
- ☐ 50 sec: Spiderman High Plank
- ☐ 10 sec: Rest
- ☐ 30 sec: Side Plank with Hip Dips (R)
- ☐ 30 sec: Side Plank with Hip Dips (L)
- ☐ 45 sec: Scorpion Push Ups
- ☐ 15 sec: Rest

4th Set: 2 Rounds
- ☐ 50 sec: Squat Thrusts
- ☐ 10 sec: Rest
- ☐ 50 sec: Alternating Jackknife Crunches
- ☐ 10 sec: Rest
- ☐ 30 sec: Wall Sit
- ☐ 30 sec: Rest

Workout #4

1st Set: 3 Rounds
- ☐ 30 sec: Sumo Squats
- ☐ 30 sec: Sumo Squat Jumps
- ☐ 30 sec: Sumo Squat Pulses
- ☐ 15 sec: Rest

2nd Set: 3 Rounds
- ☐ 30 sec: Single Leg Deadlift (R)
- ☐ 30 sec: Single Leg Deadlift (L)
- ☐ 30 sec: Fire Hydrant Kickback (R)
- ☐ 30 sec: Fire Hydrant Kickback (L)
- ☐ 15 sec: Rest

3rd Set: 3 Rounds
- ☐ 30 sec: High Plank
- ☐ 30 sec: Low Plank
- ☐ 30 sec: Plank to Push Up
- ☐ 30 sec: Low Pulsing Push Ups
- ☐ 30 sec: 1 Push Up + 8 Mountain Climbers
- ☐ 15 sec: Rest

4th Set: 2 Rounds
- ☐ 30 sec: Side Lunges
- ☐ 30 sec: Bulgarian Split Squat (R)
- ☐ 30 sec: Bulgarian Split Squat (L)
- ☐ 30 sec: Elevator Squats
- ☐ 15 sec: Rest

5th Set: 1 Round
- ☐ 60 sec: Burpee Tuck Jumps

Workout #5

1st Set: 1 Round (Warm Up)
- ☐ 2 min: Jump Rope

2nd Set: 1 Round
- ☐ 60 sec: Squats
- ☐ 60 sec: Push Ups
- ☐ 60 sec: Forward Lunges
- ☐ 60 sec: High Plank
- ☐ 60 sec: Sit Ups
- ☐ 15 sec: Rest

3rd Set: 1 Round
- ☐ 45 sec: Curtsy Squats
- ☐ 45 sec: Piked Push Ups
- ☐ 45 sec: Step Up Lunges
- ☐ 45 sec: Plank Up and Downs
- ☐ 45 sec: Cross Crunches
- ☐ 15 sec: Rest

4th Set: 1 Round
- ☐ 45 sec: In 'n Out Squats
- ☐ 45 sec: Decline Push Ups
- ☐ 45 sec: 3D Lunges
- ☐ 45 sec: Spiderman Plank
- ☐ 45 sec: Shoelace Crunches
- ☐ 15 sec: Rest

5th Set: 1 Round
- ☐ 30 sec: Squats Jacks
- ☐ 30 sec: Staggered Push Ups
- ☐ 30 sec: Lunge Burpees
- ☐ 30 sec: Low Plank Hip Twist
- ☐ 30 sec: Knees Up Crunches
- ☐ 15 sec: Rest

Workout #6

1st Set: 1 Round (Warm Up)
- ☐ 60 sec: Inchworms
- ☐ 60 sec: Cat Cows

2nd Set: 3 Rounds
- ☐ 45 sec: Horse Stance Squats
- ☐ 15 sec: Rest
- ☐ 45 sec: Rocking Tricep Dips
- ☐ 15 sec: Rest
- ☐ 30 sec: Straight Leg Hold (R)
- ☐ 30 sec: Straight Leg Hold (L)

3rd Set: 3 Rounds
- ☐ 60 sec: Alternating Squat Kicks
- ☐ 60 sec: Supermans
- ☐ 45 sec: L-Sits
- ☐ 15 sec: Rest

4th Set: 3 Rounds
- ☐ 45 sec: Pike Push Ups
- ☐ 15 sec: Rest
- ☐ 45 sec: Oblique Side Leg Raise (R)
- ☐ 45 sec: Oblique Side Leg Raise (L)
- ☐ 30 sec: Plank Back and Forths

Workout #7

1st Set: 1 Round (Warm Up)
- ☐ 90 sec: Jump Rope
- ☐ 30 sec: Downward Dog

2nd Set: 3 Rounds
- ☐ 30 sec: Squat + 2 punches
- ☐ 30 sec: Burpee Jump Over
- ☐ 30 sec: Elevator Single Leg Lunge (R)
- ☐ 30 sec: Elevator Single Leg Lunge (L)
- ☐ 30 sec: Tricep Dip Reach
- ☐ 30 sec: High Knee Run
- ☐ 15 sec: Rest

3rd Set: 2 Rounds
- ☐ 45 sec: Quick Feet
- ☐ 45 sec: Frog Burpees
- ☐ 45 sec: Sumo Squats
- ☐ 45 sec: Plank Up and Downs
- ☐ 45 sec: 3D Lunges
- ☐ 45 sec: Squat Jumps
- ☐ 45 sec: Piked Push Ups
- ☐ 15 sec: Rest

4th Set: 2 Rounds
- ☐ 45 sec: Jumping Jacks
- ☐ 45 sec: Push Up + 8 Mountain Climbers
- ☐ 45 sec: Flutter Kicks
- ☐ 45 sec: Wall Sit
- ☐ 45 sec: Low Plank with Hip Twists
- ☐ 15 sec: Rest

Workout #8

1st Set: 1 Round (Warm Up)
- ☐ 30 sec: Star Jumps
- ☐ 30 sec: Butt Kicks
- ☐ 30 sec: Switch Kick Abs
- ☐ 30 sec: Push Ups with Shoulder Taps
- ☐ 30 sec: Low Plank

2nd Set: 2 Rounds
- ☐ 45 sec: Speed Skaters
- ☐ 45 sec: Tuck Jumps
- ☐ 45 sec: Plank Toe Taps
- ☐ 45 sec: Bicycle Crunches
- ☐ 45 sec: 3D Lunges
- ☐ 15 sec: Rest

3rd Set: 3 Rounds
- ☐ 30 sec: Plank Walk Outs
- ☐ 30 sec: High Plank Alternating Leg Raise
- ☐ 30 sec: V-Ups
- ☐ 30 sec: Supermans
- ☐ 30 sec: Tricep Dips
- ☐ 30 sec: Alternating Lunge Step Ups
- ☐ 15 sec: Rest

Workout #9

1st Set: 1 Round (Warm Up)
- ☐ 60 sec: Crab Crawl
- ☐ 30 sec: Straight Leg Forward Fold
- ☐ 30 sec: Frog Pose

2nd Set: 2 Rounds
- ☐ 45 sec: Alligator Push Ups
- ☐ 15 sec: Rest
- ☐ 45 sec: Wall Sit with Calf Raise (R)
- ☐ 15 sec: Rest
- ☐ 45 sec: Wall Sit with Calf Raise (L)
- ☐ 15 sec: Rest

3rd Set: 3 Rounds
- ☐ 30 sec: X Push Ups
- ☐ 30 sec: Static V Pulses
- ☐ 30 sec: Duck Walks
- ☐ 30 sec: Mummy Sit Ups
- ☐ 30 sec: Standing Invisible Ball Twists
- ☐ 30 sec: High Knee Run
- ☐ 15 sec: Rest

4th Set: 2 Rounds
- ☐ 45 sec: Diamond Push Ups on Knees
- ☐ 15 sec: Rest
- ☐ 45 sec: Calf Raises
- ☐ 15 sec: Rest
- ☐ 45 sec: Burpee Tuck Jumps
- ☐ 15 sec: Rest

Workout #10

1st Set: 1 Round (Warm Up)
- ☐ 90 sec: Plank Walk Outs
- ☐ 30 sec: Wide Legged Forward Fold

2nd Set: 4 Rounds
- ☐ 60 sec: Speed Skaters
- ☐ 45 sec: Tricep Dips (on floor)
- ☐ 15 sec: Rest
- ☐ 45 sec: Rollercoaster Push Ups
- ☐ 15 sec: Rest

3nd Set: 4 Rounds
- ☐ 60 sec: Frog Jumps
- ☐ 45 sec: Crunchy Frogs
- ☐ 15 sec: Rest
- ☐ 45 sec: Sissy Squats
- ☐ 15 sec: Rest

4th Set: 2 Rounds
- ☐ 60 sec: Long Arm Crunch
- ☐ 30 sec: Side Crunch
- ☐ 30 sec: Side Crunch
- ☐ 10 sec: Rest

Workout #11

1st Set: 3 Rounds (Warm Up)
- ☐ 30 sec: Wall Sit
- ☐ 30 sec: Slow Push Ups

2nd Set: 2 Rounds
- ☐ 60 sec: Prisoner Squats
- ☐ 60 sec: Push Ups on Knees
- ☐ 60 sec: Calf Raises
- ☐ 60 sec: Reverse Crunches
- ☐ 15 sec: Rest

3nd Set: 2 Rounds
- ☐ 30 sec: One Leg Burpee (R)
- ☐ 30 sec: One Leg Burpee (L)
- ☐ 30 sec: Decline Push Ups
- ☐ 30 sec: Incline Push Ups
- ☐ 60 sec: Calf Raises
- ☐ 60 sec: Cross Body Crunches
- ☐ 15 sec: Rest

4th Set: 1 Round
- ☐ 60 sec: High Knee Run
- ☐ 60 sec: Low Plank

Workout #12

1st Set: 1 Round (Warm Up)
- ☐ 60 sec: Slow Burpees
- ☐ 30 sec: Pigeon Pose (R)
- ☐ 30 sec: Pigeon Pose (L)

2nd Set: 3 Rounds
- ☐ 50 sec: Good Mornings
- ☐ 10 sec: Rest
- ☐ 50 sec: Plank Walkouts
- ☐ 10 sec: Rest
- ☐ 50 sec: Diamond Push Ups from Knees
- ☐ 10 sec: Rest

3rd Set: 3 Rounds
- ☐ 40 sec: Diamond Push Ups from Knees
- ☐ 20 sec: Rest
- ☐ 40 sec: Glute Bridges
- ☐ 20 sec: Rest
- ☐ 40 sec: Step Ups
- ☐ 20 sec: Rest

4th Set: 3 Rounds
- ☐ 20 sec: Shoulder Taps
- ☐ 10 sec: Rest
- ☐ 20 sec: Cross Body Mountain Climbers
- ☐ 10 sec: Rest
- ☐ 20 sec: Tricep Dips
- ☐ 10 sec: Rest

Workout #13

1st Set: 3 Rounds
- ☐ 45 sec: Frog Jumps
- ☐ 45 sec: Jump Rope
- ☐ 45 sec: Alternating Donkey Kicks
- ☐ 45 sec: Hollow Body Hold
- ☐ 15 sec: Rest

2nd Set: 3 Rounds
- ☐ 30 sec: Forward Lunges
- ☐ 30 sec: Reverse Lunges
- ☐ 30 sec: Push Up to Down Dog
- ☐ 30 sec: Back and Forth High Plank
- ☐ 30 sec: Tuck Jumps
- ☐ 30 sec: Incline Push Ups
- ☐ 15 sec: Rest

3rd Set: 2 Rounds
- ☐ 60 sec: Floor Tuck Jumps
- ☐ 60 sec: Quick Feet
- ☐ 60 sec: Plank Up and Downs
- ☐ 15 sec: Rest

4th Set: 1 Round
- ☐ 60 sec: Burpee with Alternating Lunges

Workout #14

19

1st Set: 4 Rounds
- [ ] 60 sec: Jump Rope
- [ ] 60 sec: Alternating Reverse Lunges
- [ ] 60 sec: Low Squat Pulse
- [ ] 15 sec: Rest

2nd Set: 4 Rounds
- [ ] 60 sec: Burpees
- [ ] 60 sec: Push Ups from Knees
- [ ] 15 sec: Rest

3rd Set: 4 Rounds
- [ ] 30 sec: Glute Bridge
- [ ] 30 sec: Russian Twists
- [ ] 30 sec: Lying Straight Leg Lifts
- [ ] 30 sec: Low Plank w/ Alternating Knee Taps
- [ ] 15 sec: Rest

Workout #15

1st Set: 1 Round (Warm Up)
- ☐ 60 sec: Bear Crawl
- ☐ 30 sec: Cobra Pose
- ☐ 30 sec: Downward Dog

2nd Set: 3 Rounds
- ☐ 60 sec: Squat with Alternating Kicks
- ☐ 60 sec: Burpee with Alternating Lunges
- ☐ 60 sec: Plank with Alternating Shoulder Raise
- ☐ 15 sec: Rest

3rd Set: 3 Rounds
- ☐ 60 sec: Cross Body Mountain Climbers
- ☐ 60 sec: High Knee Run
- ☐ 30 sec: Side Plank Hip Dips (R)
- ☐ 30 sec: Side Plank Hip Dips (L)
- ☐ 15 sec: Rest

4th Set: 4 Rounds
- ☐ 30 sec: Curtsy Lunges
- ☐ 30 sec: Jump Squats
- ☐ 30 sec: Diamond Push Ups

Workout #16

1st Set: 3 Rounds
- ☐ 45 sec: Slow Squats
- ☐ 45 sec: Jump Squats
- ☐ 45 sec: Slow Push Ups
- ☐ 45 sec: Push Ups from Knees
- ☐ 15 sec: Rest

2nd Set: 3 Rounds
- ☐ 45 sec: Burpees
- ☐ 45 sec: Jumping Jacks
- ☐ 45 sec: Supermans
- ☐ 45 sec: Spiderman Push Ups
- ☐ 15 sec: Rest

3rd Set: 3 Rounds
- ☐ 30 sec: Jogging Butt Kicks
- ☐ 30 sec: Spiderman Lunges
- ☐ 30 sec: Incline Push Ups
- ☐ 15 sec: Rest

4th Set: 3 Rounds
- ☐ 40 sec: Low Plank
- ☐ 20 sec: Low Side Plank (R)
- ☐ 20 sec: Low Side Plank (L)
- ☐ 15 sec: Rest

Workout #17

1st Set: 1 Round (Warm Up)
- ☐ 45 sec: Side-to-Side Chops
- ☐ 45 sec: Straight Leg Forward Fold
- ☐ 30 sec: Frog Pose

2nd Set: 4 Rounds
- ☐ 60 sec: 2 Squat Jumps + Burpee
- ☐ 60 sec: Flutter Kicks
- ☐ 30 sec: Wide Push Ups
- ☐ 15 sec: Rest

3rd Set: 4 Rounds
- ☐ 60 sec: 2 Lunges + 1 Squat
- ☐ 60 sec: Frog Burpee + 10 Mountain Climbers
- ☐ 30 sec: Butt Kicks
- ☐ 15 sec: Rest

4th Set: 3 Rounds
- ☐ 30 sec: Speed Skaters
- ☐ 30 sec: Staggered Push Ups
- ☐ 15 sec: Rest

Workout #18

1st Set: 1 Round (Warm Up)
- ☐ 60 sec: Inchworm
- ☐ 60 sec: Forward Lunge Twists

2nd Set: 2 Rounds
- ☐ 30 sec: Jump Rope
- ☐ 30 sec: Tuck Jumps
- ☐ 30 sec: Plyometric Push Ups
- ☐ 30 sec: Runner's Skip
- ☐ 30 sec: Plank to Push Ups
- ☐ 30 sec: Low Squat Pulses
- ☐ 30 sec: Low Squat Hold
- ☐ 30 sec: Dolphin Push Ups
- ☐ 15 sec: Rest

3rd Set: 2 Rounds
- ☐ 50 sec: Clock Lunges
- ☐ 10 sec: Rest
- ☐ 50 sec: Judo Push Ups
- ☐ 10 sec: Rest
- ☐ 50 sec: Single Leg Deadlift (R)
- ☐ 10 sec: Rest
- ☐ 50 sec: Single Leg Deadlift (L)
- ☐ 10 sec: Rest
- ☐ 50 sec: Contralateral Limb Raises
- ☐ 10 sec: Rest

Workout #19

1st Set: 1 Round (Warm Up)
- ☐ 60 sec: Plank Walk Outs
- ☐ 30 sec: Side Plank (R)
- ☐ 30 sec: Side Plank (L)
- ☐ 60 sec: Downward Dog

2nd Set: 2 Rounds
- ☐ 5 Burpee Jump Overs
- ☐ 10 Frog Burpees
- ☐ 15 Long Arm Crunches
- ☐ 20 Glute Bridges
- ☐ 25 Push Ups on Knees
- ☐ 30 Pulsing Push Ups
- ☐ 35 Squats
- ☐ 40 Russian Twists (20 each side)
- ☐ 45 Flutter Kicks
- ☐ 50 High Knee Run (25 each side)

Workout #20

25

1st Set: 1 Round (Warm Up)
- ☐ 60 sec: Butt Kicks
- ☐ 30 sec: Standing Toe Taps
- ☐ 30 sec: Standing Forward Fold

2nd Set: 2 Rounds
- ☐ 30 sec: Shrimp Squats
- ☐ 30 sec: Bird Dogs
- ☐ 30 sec: YTWL
- ☐ 30 sec: Ski Hops
- ☐ 30 sec: Wall Push Ups
- ☐ 30 sec: Low Plank
- ☐ 30 sec: Rest

3rd Set: 3 Rounds
- ☐ 30 sec: Crocodile Crawl
- ☐ 30 sec: Lateral Hops
- ☐ 30 sec: Knee Slap Push Ups
- ☐ 30 sec: Single-Leg Jump Squat (R)
- ☐ 30 sec: Single-Leg Jump Squat (L)
- ☐ 30 sec: Dead Bug
- ☐ 30 sec: Rest

4th Set: 2 Rounds
- ☐ 45 sec: Quick Feet
- ☐ 15 sec: Rest
- ☐ 45 sec: Push Up + 10 mountain Climbers
- ☐ 15 sec: Rest
- ☐ 45 sec: Forward Lunges
- ☐ 15 sec: Rest

Workout #21

1st Set: 1 Round (Warm Up)
- ☐ 30 sec: Arm Circles
- ☐ 30 sec: Wall Sit
- ☐ 30 sec: Low Plank
- ☐ 30 sec: Glute Bridge Hold

2nd Set: 3 Rounds
- ☐ 45 sec: Bulgarian Split Squat (R)
- ☐ 15 sec: Rest
- ☐ 45 sec: Bulgarian Split Squat (L)
- ☐ 15 sec: Rest
- ☐ 45 sec: Twisting Sit Ups
- ☐ 15 sec: Rest
- ☐ 45 sec: Windshield Wiper Abs
- ☐ 15 sec: Rest

3rd Set: 3 Rounds
- ☐ 45 sec: Hindu Push Ups
- ☐ 15 sec: Rest
- ☐ 45 sec: Plank Toe Taps
- ☐ 15 sec: Rest
- ☐ 45 sec: Lateral Lunges
- ☐ 15 sec: Rest
- ☐ 45 sec: Jump Rope
- ☐ 15 sec: Rest

4th Set: 1 Round
- ☐ 60 sec: Jump Squats

Workout #22

1st Set: 3 Rounds (Warm Up)
- ☐ 30 sec: Downward Dog
- ☐ 30 sec: Mountain Climbers

2nd Set: 3 Rounds
- ☐ 30 sec: Star Plank
- ☐ 30 sec: Wide Push Ups
- ☐ 30 sec: Wide Push Ups From Knees
- ☐ 30 sec: Sumo Squats
- ☐ 30 sec: Sumo Squats Hold (Low)
- ☐ 30 sec: Sumo Squats Pulse (Low)
- ☐ 30 sec: Rest

3rd Set: 3 Rounds
- ☐ 30 sec: Jump Rope
- ☐ 30 sec: Jumping Jacks
- ☐ 30 sec: Jumping Lunges
- ☐ 30 sec: High Plank
- ☐ 30 sec: Floor Tuck Jumps
- ☐ 30 sec: Burpees
- ☐ 30 sec: Burpee Tuck Jumps
- ☐ 30 sec: Low Plank
- ☐ 30 sec: Rest

Workout #23

1st Set: 1 Round (Warm Up)
- [ ] 45 sec: Jump Rope
- [ ] 45 sec: Up and Down Plank
- [ ] 30 sec: Frog Pose

2nd Set: 5 Rounds
- [ ] 10 sec: Burpee Jump Over
- [ ] 20 sec: Jump Squats
- [ ] 30 sec: Diamond Push Ups
- [ ] 40 sec: Reverse Lunges
- [ ] 50 sec: Prone Back Extension
- [ ] 60 sec: Wall Sit
- [ ] 30 sec: Rest

3rd Set: 2 Rounds
- [ ] 60 sec: Slow Crunches
- [ ] 60 sec: Lying Straight Leg Raises
- [ ] 60 sec: Bicycle Crunches

Workout #24

1st Set: 1 Round (Warm Up)
- ☐ 45 sec: Jump Rope
- ☐ 45 sec: Cross Body Mountain Climbers
- ☐ 30 sec: Cat Cows

2nd Set: 4 Rounds
- ☐ 40 sec: Speed Skaters
- ☐ 20 sec: Rest
- ☐ 40 sec: Squat with Front Kicks
- ☐ 20 sec: Rest
- ☐ 40 sec: Staggered Push Ups
- ☐ 20 sec: Rest
- ☐ 40 sec: Low Plank with Lateral Punches
- ☐ 20 sec: Rest
- ☐ 40 sec: Glute Bridges
- ☐ 20 sec: Rest

3rd Set: 3 Rounds
- ☐ 30 sec: Standing Mountain Climbers
- ☐ 30 sec: Frog Burpees
- ☐ 30 sec: Spiderman Push Ups
- ☐ 30 sec: Rest

Workout #25

1st Set: 1 Rounds (Warm Up)
- ☐ 60 sec: Happy Baby Pose
- ☐ 60 sec: Slow Bicycle Crunches

2nd Set: 4 Rounds
- ☐ 15 Triple-Pulse Jump Squats
- ☐ 20 Squat with Overhead Press
- ☐ 15 Bulgarian Squats (R)
- ☐ 15 Bulgarian Squats (L)
- ☐ 30 sec: Rest

3rd Set: 2 Rounds
- ☐ 15 (each side) Oblique Plank Twist
- ☐ 15 Plank Walk Outs
- ☐ 30 sec: Rest

4th Set: 4 Rounds
- ☐ 20 Box Jump with Double Squats
- ☐ 20 Pike Push Ups
- ☐ 15 Spiderman Plank Crunch
- ☐ 10 (each side) Side Plank with Hip Dips
- ☐ 30 sec: Rest

Workout #26

1st Set: 2 Rounds (Warm Up)
- ☐ 30 sec: 3D Lunges
- ☐ 30 sec: High Plank
- ☐ 30 sec: Slow Push Ups
- ☐ 30 sec: Supermans

2nd Set: 4 Rounds
- ☐ 60 sec: Elevated Squats
- ☐ 60 sec: Deep Jump Squats
- ☐ 60 sec: Hip Thrusts
- ☐ 60 sec: Plyometric Bench Hops
- ☐ 60 sec: Low Plank Alternating Side Punches
- ☐ 30 sec: Rest

3rd Set: 2 Rounds
- ☐ 45 sec: Wide Push Ups from Knees
- ☐ 45 sec: Diamond Push Ups from Knees
- ☐ 30 sec: Rest

Workout #27

1st Set: 1 Round (Warm Up)
- ☐ 60 sec: Bear Crawls
- ☐ 30 sec: Standing Side Bend (R)
- ☐ 30 sec: Standing Side Bend (L)

2nd Set: 3 Rounds
- ☐ 45 sec: Single Leg Glute Bridge (R)
- ☐ 15 sec: Rest
- ☐ 45 sec: Single Leg Glute Bridge (L)
- ☐ 15 sec: Rest
- ☐ 45 sec: Box Jumps
- ☐ 15 sec: Rest

3rd Set: 3 Rounds
- ☐ 45 sec: Side Plank with Leg Lifts (R)
- ☐ 15 sec: Rest
- ☐ 45 sec: Side Plank with Leg Lifts (L)
- ☐ 15 sec: Rest
- ☐ 45 sec: Roller Coaster Push Ups
- ☐ 15 sec: Rest

4th Set: 2 Rounds
- ☐ 30 sec: Negative Push Ups
- ☐ 30 sec: Pistol Squats
- ☐ 30 sec: Bench Dips

Workout #28

1st Set: 1 Round (Warm Up)
- [ ] 60 sec: Jump Rope
- [ ] 60 sec: Lying Windshield Wipers

2nd Set: 5 Rounds
- [ ] 25 sec: Frankenstein Kicks
- [ ] 25 sec: Jump Squats
- [ ] 10 sec: Rest

3rd Set: 5 Rounds
- [ ] 25 sec: Low Plank
- [ ] 25 sec: Push Ups on Knees
- [ ] 10 sec: Rest

4th Set: 5 Rounds
- [ ] 25 sec: Wall Sit
- [ ] 25 sec: Jumping Lunges
- [ ] 10 sec: Rest

5th Set: 5 Rounds
- [ ] 25 sec: Isometric Push Ups
- [ ] 25 sec: Cross Body Mountain Climbers
- [ ] 10 sec: Rest

Workout #29

1st Set: 1 Round (Warm Up)
- ☐ 45 sec: Arm Circles
- ☐ 45 sec: Hip Openers
- ☐ 30 sec: High Plank

2nd Set: 3 Rounds
- ☐ 60 sec: Jump Rope
- ☐ 45 sec: Alternating Donkey Kicks
- ☐ 15 sec: Rest
- ☐ 60 sec: Plank Shoulder Taps
- ☐ 45 sec: Frog Burpees
- ☐ 15 sec: Rest
- ☐ 60 sec: Forward Lunges
- ☐ 45 sec: Push Up Jacks
- ☐ 15 sec: Rest
- ☐ 60 sec: Plank Toe Taps
- ☐ 45 sec: High Knee Run
- ☐ 15 sec: Rest
- ☐ 60 sec: Bird Dogs
- ☐ 45 sec: Alternating Heel Touches

Workout #30

1st Set: 1 Round (Warm Up)
- ☐ 60 sec: Alternating Lateral Lunge with Reach
- ☐ 30 sec: Wide Legged Forward Fold
- ☐ 30 sec: Low Plank

2nd Set: 2 Rounds
- ☐ 45 sec: Lateral Jumps
- ☐ 45 sec: Inchworms
- ☐ 45 sec: Tuck Jumps
- ☐ 45 sec: Calf Raises
- ☐ 15 sec: Rest

3rd Set: 2 Rounds
- ☐ 30 sec: Speed Skaters
- ☐ 30 sec: Butt Kicks
- ☐ 30 sec: Wall Sit
- ☐ 30 sec: Plank Jacks
- ☐ 15 sec: Rest

4th Set: 2 Rounds
- ☐ 45 sec: Push Ups with Alternating Shoulder Raise
- ☐ 45 sec: Side Oblique Crunch (R)
- ☐ 45 sec: Side Oblique Crunch (L)
- ☐ 45 sec: Flutter Kicks
- ☐ 15 sec: Rest

5th Set: 2 Rounds
- ☐ 25 sec: Frog Sit Ups
- ☐ 25 sec: Russian Twists
- ☐ 10 sec: Rest

Workout #31

1st Set: 1 Round (Warm Up)
- ☐ 60 sec: Squat to Raised Heel
- ☐ 60 sec: Downward Dog
- ☐ 60 sec: Cat Cows

2nd Set: 1 Round
- ☐ 50 sec: Prone Walk Out
- ☐ 10 sec: Rest
- ☐ 50 sec: Dead Bugs
- ☐ 10 sec: Rest
- ☐ 50 sec: Frog Push Ups
- ☐ 10 sec: Rest
- ☐ 50 sec: Alternating Side Lunges
- ☐ 10 sec: Rest

3rd Set: 2 Rounds
- ☐ 40 sec: Knee to Elbow Push Ups
- ☐ 20 sec: Low Plank
- ☐ 40 sec: Squat with Alternating Kicks
- ☐ 20 sec: Wall Sit
- ☐ 40 sec: Burpees
- ☐ 20 sec: Supermans
- ☐ 40 sec: Russian Twists
- ☐ 20 sec: Lying Leg Lifts

4th Set: 3 Rounds
- ☐ 30 sec: Lying Leg Lifts (R)
- ☐ 30 sec: Lying Leg Lifts (L)
- ☐ 30 sec: High Plank Shoulder Taps (R)
- ☐ 30 sec: High Plank Shoulder Taps (L)
- ☐ 30 sec: Single Leg Glute Bridge (R)
- ☐ 30 sec: Single Leg Glute Bridge (L)
- ☐ 30 sec: Low Plank Side Punches (R)
- ☐ 30 sec: Low Plank Side Punches (L)

Workout #32

1st Set: 1 Round (Warm Up)
- ☐ 45 sec: Squat to Overhead Reach
- ☐ 45 sec: Jumping Jacks
- ☐ 30 sec: Frog Pose

2nd Set: 4 Rounds
- ☐ 50 sec: Bicycle Crunches
- ☐ 10 sec: Rest
- ☐ 50 sec: Cross Body Mountain Climbers
- ☐ 10 sec: Rest
- ☐ 30 sec: One Legged Deadlifts (R)
- ☐ 30 sec: One Legged Deadlifts (L)
- ☐ 50 sec: Push Ups from Knees
- ☐ 10 sec: Rest
- ☐ 50 sec: In-n-Out Squats
- ☐ 10 sec: Rest
- ☐ 30 sec: Side Plank with Leg Lift (R)
- ☐ 30 sec: Side Plank with Leg Lift (L)
- ☐ 50 sec: Burpees
- ☐ 10 sec: Rest

Workout #33

1st Set: 1 Round (Warm Up)
- ☐ 30 sec: Half Jacks
- ☐ 30 sec: Torso Rotations
- ☐ 60 sec: Straight Leg Forward Fold

2nd Set: 2 Rounds
- ☐ 30 sec: Decline Push Ups
- ☐ 30 sec: Bench Dips
- ☐ 30 sec: Low Plank with Alternating Knee Taps
- ☐ 30 sec: High Plank with Alternating Shoulder Raises
- ☐ 30 sec: Rest

3rd Set: 3 Rounds
- ☐ 45 sec: Alternating Turning Kicks
- ☐ 45 sec: Squat with Alternating Knee Lift
- ☐ 45 sec: Overhead Forward Lunges
- ☐ 45 sec: Squat + 2 Reverse Lunges
- ☐ 30 sec: Low Squat Hold

4th Set: 3 Rounds
- ☐ 45 sec: Tricep Dip Reach
- ☐ 45 sec: Elevator Push Ups
- ☐ 45 sec: Shoelace Crunches
- ☐ 45 sec: Push Up + 8 Mountain Climbers
- ☐ 45 sec: Uppercut Punches
- ☐ 45 sec: Side Chops
- ☐ 30 sec: High Plank

Workout #34

1st Set: 1 Round (Warm Up)
- ☐ 60 sec: Inchworms
- ☐ 60 sec: Push Ups from Knees
- ☐ 60 sec: Slow Squats

2nd Set: 4 Rounds
- ☐ 20 sec: Close Squat Jumps
- ☐ 10 sec: Rest
- ☐ 20 sec: Plank Jump In-n-Outs
- ☐ 10 sec: Rest

3rd Set: 4 Rounds
- ☐ 20 sec: Reverse Lunges with Knee Drive
- ☐ 10 sec: Rest
- ☐ 20 sec: Mountain Climbers
- ☐ 10 sec: Rest

4th Set: 4 Rounds
- ☐ 20 sec: Speed Skaters
- ☐ 10 sec: Rest
- ☐ 20 sec: High Knee Run
- ☐ 10 sec: Rest

5th Set: 4 Rounds
- ☐ 20 sec: Pike Push Ups
- ☐ 10 sec: Rest
- ☐ 20 sec: Up and Down Planks
- ☐ 10 sec: Rest

Workout #35

1st Set: 1 Round (Warm Up)
- ☐ 30 sec: Bird Dogs (L)
- ☐ 30 sec: Bird Dogs (R)
- ☐ 60 sec: Downward Dog Push Ups

2nd Set: 2 Rounds
- ☐ 30 sec: Diamond Push Ups
- ☐ 30 sec: Low Side Plank (R)
- ☐ 30 sec: Wide Push Ups
- ☐ 30 sec: Low Side Plank (L)
- ☐ 30 sec: Rest

3rd Set: 2 Rounds
- ☐ 30 sec: Lying Single Leg Hold (R)
- ☐ 30 sec: Lying Single Leg Hold (L)
- ☐ 30 sec: Switch Kick Abs
- ☐ 30 sec: Bicycle Crunches
- ☐ 30 sec: Rest

4th Set: 2 Rounds
- ☐ 30 sec: Bulgarian Squats (R)
- ☐ 30 sec: Bulgarian Squats (L)
- ☐ 30 sec: Alternating Lateral Lunges
- ☐ 30 sec: Reverse Lunges
- ☐ 30 sec: Jump Squats
- ☐ 30 sec: Burpees
- ☐ 30 sec: Rest

Workout #36

41

1st Set: 1 Round (Warm Up)
- ☐ 60 sec: Frankenstein Kicks
- ☐ 60 sec: Arm Circles

2nd Set: 4 Rounds
- ☐ 20 Fast Air Squats
- ☐ 15 Curtsy Lunges (15 each side)
- ☐ 30 High Plank Jacks
- ☐ 60 Forward Lunges
- ☐ 20 Mountain Climbers (10 each side)
- ☐ 30 sec: Rest

3rd Set: 4 Rounds
- ☐ 20 Fast Push Ups
- ☐ 15 Plank to Push Ups
- ☐ 30 sec: Low Plank
- ☐ 60 sec: Supermans
- ☐ 20 Crossing Mountain Climbers (10 each side)
- ☐ 30 sec: Rest

Workout #37

1st Set: 1 Round (Warm Up)
- ☐ 60 sec: Downward Dog
- ☐ 30 sec: One Legged Mountain Climbers (R)
- ☐ 30 sec: One Legged Mountain Climbers (L)

2nd Set: 5 Rounds
- ☐ 30 sec: Bulgarian Squats (R)
- ☐ 30 sec: Bulgarian Squats (L)
- ☐ 30 sec: Alternating Lateral Lunges
- ☐ 30 sec: Reverse Lunges
- ☐ 30 sec: Jump Squats
- ☐ 30 sec: High Plank
- ☐ 30 sec: Burpees
- ☐ 30 sec: Rest

3rd Set: 2 Rounds
- ☐ 20 High Plank Jacks
- ☐ 20 Jumping Lunges (10 each side)
- ☐ 20 Wide Push Ups
- ☐ 20 Supermans

Workout #38

1st Set: 3 Rounds (Warm Up)
- ☐ 30 sec: High Knee Run + Cross Body Punches
- ☐ 30 sec: Slow Push Ups

2nd Set: 3 Rounds
- ☐ 30 sec: Squat with Leg Kick (R)
- ☐ 30 sec: Squat with Leg Kick (L)
- ☐ 30 sec: Pike Push Ups
- ☐ 30 sec: Low Plank
- ☐ 30 sec: Standing Quick Feet
- ☐ 30 sec: Rest

3rd Set: 3 Rounds
- ☐ 30 sec: Squat with 2 Cross Punches
- ☐ 30 sec: Low Squat Pulses
- ☐ 30 sec: Plank Jacks
- ☐ 30 sec: T Plank
- ☐ 30 sec: Russian Twists
- ☐ 30 sec: Rest

4th Set: 3 Rounds
- ☐ 30 sec: Mountain Climber Knee to Elbow (R)
- ☐ 30 sec: Mountain Climber Knee to Elbow (L)
- ☐ 30 sec: Star Jumps
- ☐ 30 sec: Plank Shoulder Taps
- ☐ 30 sec: Prisoner Squats
- ☐ 30 sec: Rest

Workout #39

1st Set: 2 Rounds (Warm Up)
- ☐ 30 sec: Lateral Leg Swings (L)
- ☐ 30 sec: Lateral Leg Swings (R)
- ☐ 30 sec: High Plank

2nd Set: 2 Rounds
- ☐ 45 sec: Push Up Jack with Shoulder Taps
- ☐ 15 sec: Rest
- ☐ 45 sec: Slow Lying Straight Leg Lifts
- ☐ 15 sec: Rest
- ☐ 45 sec: Standing Switch Kick Punch
- ☐ 15 sec: Rest
- ☐ 45 sec: Heel Elevated Squats
- ☐ 15 sec: Rest

3rd Set: 2 Rounds
- ☐ 45 sec: Roller Coaster Push Ups
- ☐ 15 sec: Rest
- ☐ 45 sec: Sumo Squats
- ☐ 15 sec: Rest
- ☐ 45 sec: Low Side Plank Hip Dips (L)
- ☐ 15 sec: Rest
- ☐ 45 sec: Low Side Plank Hip Dips (R)
- ☐ 15 sec: Rest

4th Set: 3 Rounds
- ☐ 30 sec: Spider Lunges (L)
- ☐ 30 sec: Spider Lunges (R)
- ☐ 30 sec: Slow Wide Push Ups
- ☐ 30 sec: Plank Toe Taps (L)
- ☐ 30 sec: Plank Toe Taps (R)
- ☐ 30 sec: Rest

5th Set: 1 Round
- ☐ 60 sec: Burpees with Alternating Lunges

Workout #40

45

1st Set: 1 Round (Warm Up)
- ☐ 60 sec: Standing Mountain Climbers
- ☐ 60 sec: Cat Cows

2nd Set: 4 Rounds
- ☐ 30 sec: Undercut Punches with Wide Bent Knees
- ☐ 30 sec: Push Up with Alternating Side Punches
- ☐ 30 sec: In-n-Out Abs
- ☐ 30 sec: Rest

3rd Set: 2 Rounds
- ☐ 45 sec: Squat with Alternating Side Leg Lifts
- ☐ 15 sec: Rest
- ☐ 45 sec: Wide Pike Push Ups
- ☐ 15 sec: Rest
- ☐ 45 sec: Fast Jumping Jacks
- ☐ 15 sec: Rest

4th Set: 4 Rounds
- ☐ 30 sec: Ski Hops
- ☐ 30 sec: Alternating Staggered Push Ups
- ☐ 30 sec: Switch Kick Abs
- ☐ 30 sec: Rest

5th Set: 2 Rounds
- ☐ 20 sec: Squat with Alternating Oblique Crunch
- ☐ 10 sec: Rest
- ☐ 20 sec: Plank with Alternating Oblique Crunch
- ☐ 10 sec: Rest
- ☐ 20 sec: Push Up with Alternating Oblique Crunch
- ☐ 10 sec: Rest

Workout #41

1st Set: 1 Round (Warm Up)
- ☐ 60 sec: Jog in Place
- ☐ 60 sec: Pigeon Pose (R)
- ☐ 60 sec: Pigeon Pose (L)

2nd Set: 3 Rounds
- ☐ 12 Squats (3 sec down, 1 sec up)
- ☐ 15 Bulgarian Squat (R)
- ☐ 15 Bulgarian Squat (L)
- ☐ 12 Sumo Squats (3 sec down, 1 sec up)
- ☐ 30 sec: Wall Sit

3rd Set: 3 Rounds
- ☐ 12 Push Ups (3 sec down, 1 sec up)
- ☐ 15 Side Plank Hip Dips (R)
- ☐ 15 Side Plank Hip Dips (L)
- ☐ 12 Bench Dips (3 sec down, 1 sec up)
- ☐ 30 sec: Low Push Up Pulses

4th Set: 2 Rounds
- ☐ 30 sec: Speed Skaters
- ☐ 30 sec: Jump Rope
- ☐ 30 sec: Burpee Jump Overs
- ☐ 30 sec: Knees Up Crunches

Workout #42

47

1st Set: 2 Rounds (Warm Up)
- [ ] 30 sec: High Plank
- [ ] 30 sec: High Plank In-n-Outs

2nd Set: 3 Rounds
- [ ] 15 Reverse Lunge to Forward Kicks (R)
- [ ] 15 Reverse Lunge to Forward Kicks (L)
- [ ] 10 Bird Dog Crunch (10 each side)
- [ ] 12 Plyo Push Ups
- [ ] 30 Lying Straight Leg Cross Punches (15 each side)

3rd Set: 3 Rounds
- [ ] 10 Box Jumps
- [ ] 15 Supermans
- [ ] 10 Diamond Push Ups
- [ ] 15 Elevator Squats
- [ ] 40 Heel Touching Crunches (20 each side)

4th Set: 2 Rounds
- [ ] 45 sec: Frog Jumps
- [ ] 15 sec: Rest
- [ ] 45 sec: Decline Push Ups
- [ ] 15 sec: Rest

Workout #43

1st Set: 1 Round (Warm Up)
- ☐ 60 sec: Walkout with Lunge and Twist
- ☐ 60 sec: Push Ups from Knees

2nd Set: 3 Rounds
- ☐ 30 sec: Standing Switch Kicks
- ☐ 30 sec: Butt Kicks with Arms Overhead
- ☐ 30 sec: Power Knees (R)
- ☐ 30 sec: Power Knees (L)
- ☐ 30 sec: Rest

3rd Set: 4 Rounds
- ☐ 20 sec: Power Jacks
- ☐ 10 sec: Rest
- ☐ 20 sec: Push Up Jacks
- ☐ 10 sec: Rest
- ☐ 20 sec: Low Plank with Oblique Crunch (R)
- ☐ 10 sec: Rest
- ☐ 20 sec: Low Plank with Oblique Crunch (L)
- ☐ 10 sec: Rest

4th Set: 2 Rounds
- ☐ 50 sec: Globe Jumps
- ☐ 10 sec: Rest
- ☐ 50 sec: High Plank Toe Taps
- ☐ 10 sec: Rest
- ☐ 50 sec: Flutter Kicks
- ☐ 10 sec: Rest

Workout #44

49

1st Set: 1 Round (Warm Up)
- ☐ 45 sec: Hip Openers
- ☐ 45 sec: Chest Openers
- ☐ 30 sec: Neck Rotations

2nd Set: 2 Rounds
- ☐ 15 Slow Push Ups
- ☐ 15 Slow Squats
- ☐ 15 Slow Split Leg Lunge (R)
- ☐ 15 Slow Split Leg Lunge (L)
- ☐ 15 Slow Crunches

3rd Set: 5 Rounds
- ☐ 30 sec: Frog Burpees
- ☐ 30 sec: High Plank Shoulder Taps
- ☐ 30 sec: High Knees with Arms Overhead
- ☐ 30 sec: Sit Up Punches
- ☐ 30 sec: Rest

4th Set: 2 Rounds
- ☐ 10 Slow Push Ups
- ☐ 10 Slow Squats
- ☐ 10 Slow Split Leg Lunge (R)
- ☐ 10 Slow Split Leg Lunge (L)
- ☐ 10 Slow Crunches

Workout #45

1st Set: 1 Round (Warm Up)
- ☐ 60 sec: Inchworms
- ☐ 60 sec: Low Plank Hip Twists

2nd Set: 1 Round
- ☐ 10 Burpees
- ☐ 10 Frog Burpees
- ☐ 10 Burpee Jacks
- ☐ 10 Burpee Tuck Jumps

3rd Set: 2 Rounds
- ☐ 20 Wide Push Ups
- ☐ 20 Supermans
- ☐ 20 Diamond Push Ups
- ☐ 20 High Plank with Front Shoulder Raise (10 each side)

4th Set: 3 Rounds
- ☐ 30 Air Squats
- ☐ 30 Reverse Lunge with Forward Kick (15 each side)
- ☐ 30 Jump Squats
- ☐ 30 Jumping Lunges (15 each side)

5th Set: 4 Rounds
- ☐ 40 Crunches
- ☐ 40 Bicycle Crunches (20 each side)
- ☐ 40 Shoelace Crunches
- ☐ 40 Switch Kick Abs (20 each side)

Workout #46

1st Set: 1 Round (Warm Up)
- ☐ 60 sec: Alternating Bird Dogs
- ☐ 60 sec: Jump Rope

2nd Set: 3 Round
- ☐ 50 sec: Sumo Squat Jumps
- ☐ 10 sec: Rest
- ☐ 50 sec: Plyo Push Ups From Knees
- ☐ 10 sec: Rest
- ☐ 50 sec: Low Plank Hip Twists
- ☐ 10 sec: Rest

3rd Set: 3 Rounds
- ☐ 50 sec: Wall Sit with Heels Elevated
- ☐ 10 sec: Rest
- ☐ 50 sec: Roller Coasters
- ☐ 10 sec: Rest
- ☐ 50 sec: Low Plank with Alternating Knee Taps
- ☐ 10 sec: Rest

4th Set: 3 Rounds
- ☐ 20 Fire Hydrants (R)
- ☐ 20 Fire Hydrants (L)
- ☐ 30 Low Squat Pulses

Workout #47

1st Set: 1 Round (Warm Up)
- ☐ 60 sec: Alternating Bird Dogs
- ☐ 60 sec: Jump Rope

2nd Set: 3 Round
- ☐ 50 sec: Sumo Squat Jumps
- ☐ 10 sec: Rest
- ☐ 50 sec: Plyo Push Ups From Knees
- ☐ 10 sec: Rest
- ☐ 50 sec: Low Plank Hip Twists
- ☐ 10 sec: Rest

3rd Set: 3 Rounds
- ☐ 50 sec: Wall Sit with Heels Elevated
- ☐ 10 sec: Rest
- ☐ 50 sec: Roller Coasters
- ☐ 10 sec: Rest
- ☐ 50 sec: Low Plank with Alternating Knee Taps
- ☐ 10 sec: Rest

4th Set: 3 Rounds
- ☐ 20 Fire Hydrants (R)
- ☐ 20 Fire Hydrants (L)
- ☐ 30 Low Squat Pulses
- ☐ 50 Calf Raises

Workout #48

1st Set: 1 Round (Warm Up)
- ☐ 45 sec: Groiners
- ☐ 45 sec: Spider Crawl
- ☐ 45 sec: Standing Long Jump

2nd Set: 3 Round
- ☐ 25 Squats
- ☐ 25 Push Ups
- ☐ 50 Lunges (25 each side)
- ☐ 10 Pike Push Ups
- ☐ 25 In-n-Out Abs
- ☐ 60 sec: Plank

3rd Set: 3 Rounds
- ☐ 45 sec: Hollow Rocks
- ☐ 15 sec: Rest
- ☐ 45 sec: Slow Tuck Jumps
- ☐ 15 sec: Rest
- ☐ 45 sec: Tricep Dips
- ☐ 15 sec: Rest

Workout #49

1st Set: 1 Round (Warm Up)
- ☐ 60 sec: Bear Crawl

2nd Set: 1 Round
- ☐ 10 Burpees, 10 Mountain Climbers, 10 Sit Ups
- ☐ 9 Burpees, 9 Mountain Climbers, 9 Sit Ups
- ☐ 8 Burpees, 8 Mountain Climbers, 8 Sit Ups
- ☐ 7 Burpees, 7 Mountain Climbers, 7 Sit Ups
- ☐ 6 Burpees, 6 Mountain Climbers, 6 Sit Ups
- ☐ 5 Burpees, 5 Mountain Climbers, 5 Sit Ups
- ☐ 4 Burpees, 4 Mountain Climbers, 4 Sit Ups
- ☐ 3 Burpees, 3 Mountain Climbers, 3 Sit Ups
- ☐ 2 Burpees, 2 Mountain Climbers, 2 Sit Ups
- ☐ 1 Burpees, 1 Mountain Climbers, 1 Sit Ups

3rd Set: 3 Rounds
- ☐ 30 sec: Dragon Walk
- ☐ 30 sec: One Legged Glute Bridge (R)
- ☐ 30 sec: One Legged Glute Bridge (L)
- ☐ 30 sec: Russian Twists

Workout #50

55

1st Set: 1 Round (Warm Up)
- [ ] 30 sec: Low Plank
- [ ] 30 sec: Push Ups

2nd Set: 2 Rounds
- [ ] 60 sec: Jump Lunges
- [ ] 30 sec: Side Plank with Leg Lift (R)
- [ ] 30 sec: Side Plank with Leg Lift (L)
- [ ] 60 sec: Supermans

3rd Set: 1 Round
- [ ] 20 Push Ups, 1 Squat
- [ ] 19 Push Ups, 2 Squats
- [ ] 18 Push Ups, 3 Squats
- [ ] 17 Push Ups, 4 Squats
- [ ] 16 Push Ups, 5 Squats
- [ ] 15 Push Ups, 6 Squats
- [ ] 14 Push Ups, 7 Squats
- [ ] 13 Push Ups, 8 Squats
- [ ] 12 Push Ups, 9 Squats
- [ ] 11 Push Ups, 10 Squats
- [ ] 10 Push Ups, 11 Squats
- [ ] 9 Push Ups, 12 Squats
- [ ] 8 Push Ups, 13 Squats
- [ ] 7 Push Ups, 14 Squats
- [ ] 6 Push Ups, 15 Squats
- [ ] 5 Push Ups, 16 Squats
- [ ] 4 Push Ups, 17 Squats
- [ ] 3 Push Ups, 18 Squats
- [ ] 2 Push Ups, 19 Squats

Workout #51

1st Set: 1 Round (Warm Up)
- ☐ 60 sec: Frankenstein Kicks

2nd Set: 5 Rounds
- ☐ 24 Sumo Squats
- ☐ 24 Wide Push Ups
- ☐ 24 Curtsy Lunges (12 each side)
- ☐ 60 sec: Jump Rope

3rd Set: 3 Rounds
- ☐ 20 sec: V-Ups
- ☐ 10 sec: Rest
- ☐ 20 sec: Cross Crunches
- ☐ 10 sec: Rest
- ☐ 20 sec: Low Plank
- ☐ 10 sec: Rest

Workout #52

1st Set: 1 Round (Warm Up)
- ☐ 60 sec: Jumping Jacks

2nd Set: 2 Rounds
- ☐ 10 Burpees
- ☐ 60 sec: High Knee Run
- ☐ 10 Squats
- ☐ 60 sec: Butt Kicks
- ☐ 10 Push Ups
- ☐ 60 sec: Speed Skaters
- ☐ 10 Sit Ups
- ☐ 60 sec: Jump Rope

3rd Set: 2 Rounds
- ☐ 20 Frog Burpees
- ☐ 30 sec: High Knee Run
- ☐ 20 Close Squats
- ☐ 30 sec: Butt Kicks
- ☐ 20 Diamond Push Ups
- ☐ 30 sec: Speed Skaters
- ☐ 20 Scissor Kicks
- ☐ 30 sec: Jump Rope

Workout #53

1st Set: 1 Round (Warm Up)
- ☐ 60 sec: Downward Dog

2nd Set: 25 Rounds
- ☐ 1 Burpee
- ☐ 1 Push Up
- ☐ 1 Squat
- ☐ 1 Jumping Jack
- ☐ 1 Sit Up

3rd Set: 3 Rounds
- ☐ 45 sec: High Knee Run with Cross Punches
- ☐ 15 sec: Rest
- ☐ 45 sec: Plank Jacks
- ☐ 15 sec: Rest

Workout #54

1st Set: 1 Round (Warm Up)
- ☐ 60 sec: Forward Lunges with Torso Twist

2nd Set: 3 Rounds
- ☐ 20 Squats
- ☐ 20 Reverse Lunges
- ☐ 10 Squat Jumps
- ☐ 20 Jumping Lunges

3rd Set: 3 Rounds
- ☐ 20 Push Ups
- ☐ 20 Bench Dips
- ☐ 10 Slow Push Ups
- ☐ 20 Tricep Dip Reach

4th Set: 1 Round
- ☐ 60 sec: Lying Leg Raises
- ☐ 30 sec: Lying Leg Hold (R)
- ☐ 30 sec: Lying Leg Hold (L)
- ☐ 60 sec: Reverse Crunches

Workout #55

1st Set: 1 Round (Warm Up)
- ☐ 60 sec: Lateral Lunges
- ☐ 60 sec: High Plank

2nd Set: 10 Rounds
- ☐ 4 Overhead Squats
- ☐ 4 Jumping Lunges
- ☐ 4 Supermans
- ☐ 4 Sit Ups

3rd Set: 10 Rounds
- ☐ 4 Staggered Push Ups
- ☐ 4 Roller Coasters
- ☐ 4 Side Plank Hip Dips (R)
- ☐ 4 Side Plank Hip Dips (L)

4th Set: 3 Rounds
- ☐ 30 sec: Glute Bridge Hold
- ☐ 30 sec: Diamond Sit Ups
- ☐ 30 sec: Plank Rotations
- ☐ 30 sec: Pulsing Push Ups

Workout #56

1st Set: 1 Round (Warm Up)
- [ ] 60 sec: Slow Mountain Climbers
- [ ] 30 sec: Arm Circles

2nd Set: 2 Rounds
- [ ] 20 Burpees
- [ ] 40 Reverse Lunges (20 each side)
- [ ] 60 sec: High Knee Run
- [ ] 20 Push Ups
- [ ] 40 Forward Lunges (20 each side)
- [ ] 60 sec: High Knee Run
- [ ] 20 Supermans
- [ ] 40 Lateral Lunges (20 each side)
- [ ] 60 sec: Wall Sit

3rd Set: 3 Rounds
- [ ] 30 sec: Donkey Kicks (R)
- [ ] 30 sec: Donkey Kicks (L)
- [ ] 30 sec: Side Plank (R)
- [ ] 30 sec: Side Plank (L)

Workout #57

62

1st Set: 1 Round (Warm Up)
- ☐ 60 sec: Child's Pose
- ☐ 60 sec: Downward Dog

2nd Set: 2 Rounds
- ☐ 50 Plank Knee Taps
- ☐ 40 Push Ups
- ☐ 30 Jumping Lunges
- ☐ 20 Shoelace Crunches
- ☐ 10 Bench Dips
- ☐ 40 Hip Lift Crunches
- ☐ 30 Push Ups
- ☐ 20 Jump Squats
- ☐ 10 Bird Dogs + Knee Touch (5 each side)
- ☐ 30 Flutter Kicks
- ☐ 20 Plyo Push Ups
- ☐ 10 Burpees

Workout #58

1st Set: 1 Round (Warm Up)
- ☐ 60 sec: Inchworms

2nd Set: 10 Rounds
- ☐ 20 Cross Body Mountain Climbers
- ☐ 20 Heel Touch Crunches
- ☐ 20 Squats
- ☐ 20 Push Ups

3rd Set: 3 Rounds
- ☐ 20 sec: High Knee Run
- ☐ 10 sec: Rest
- ☐ 20 sec: Butt Kicks
- ☐ 10 sec: Rest
- ☐ 20 sec: Speed Skaters
- ☐ 10 sec: Rest

Workout #59

1st Set: 1 Round (Warm Up)
- ☐ 60 sec: Inchworms

2nd Set: 1 Round
- ☐ 20 Burpees, 1 Sit Up
- ☐ 19 Burpees, 2 Sit Ups
- ☐ 18 Burpees, 3 Sit Ups
- ☐ 17 Burpees, 4 Sit Ups
- ☐ 16 Burpees, 5 Sit Ups
- ☐ 15 Burpees, 6 Sit Ups
- ☐ 14 Burpees, 7 Sit Ups
- ☐ 13 Burpees, 8 Sit Ups
- ☐ 12 Burpees, 9 Sit Ups
- ☐ 11 Burpees, 10 Sit Ups
- ☐ 10 Burpees, 11 Sit Ups
- ☐ 9 Burpees, 12 Sit Ups
- ☐ 8 Burpees, 13 Sit Ups
- ☐ 7 Burpees, 14 Sit Ups
- ☐ 6 Burpees, 15 Sit Ups
- ☐ 5 Burpees, 16 Sit Ups
- ☐ 4 Burpees, 17 Sit Ups
- ☐ 3 Burpees, 18 Sit Ups
- ☐ 2 Burpees, 19 Sit Ups
- ☐ 1 Burpee, 20 Sit Ups

Workout #60

1st Set: 1 Round (Warm Up)
- ☐ 60 sec: Inchworms

2nd Set: 5 Rounds
- ☐ 10 Squat with Alternating Front Kick
- ☐ 10 Reverse Lunges (R)
- ☐ 10 Reverse Lunges (L)
- ☐ 10 Glute Bridge

3rd Set: 5 Rounds
- ☐ 10 Push Up with 2 Shoulder Taps
- ☐ 10 Side Plank Hip Dips (R)
- ☐ 10 Side Plank Hip Dips (L)
- ☐ 10 Supermans

4th Set: 5 Rounds
- ☐ 10 Cross Punch Sit Ups
- ☐ 10 Lying Leg Lifts
- ☐ 10 Frog Crunches
- ☐ 5 Burpees

Workout #61

1st Set: 1 Round (Warm Up)
- ☐ 60 sec: V-Ups

2nd Set: 3 Rounds
- ☐ 20 sec: Burpee Lunges
- ☐ 10 sec: Rest
- ☐ 20 sec: Single Leg Lunge Jump (R)
- ☐ 10 sec: Rest
- ☐ 20 sec: Single Leg Lunge Jump (L)
- ☐ 10 sec: Rest
- ☐ 20 sec: Single Leg Lunge Hold (R)
- ☐ 10 sec: Rest
- ☐ 20 sec: Single Leg Lunge Hold (L)
- ☐ 10 sec: Rest

3rd Set: 3 Rounds
- ☐ 20 sec: Staggered Push Ups
- ☐ 10 sec: Rest
- ☐ 20 sec: Plyo Push Ups from Knees
- ☐ 10 sec: Rest
- ☐ 20 sec: Push Up Rows
- ☐ 10 sec: Rest
- ☐ 20 sec: Low Push Up Hold
- ☐ 10 sec: Rest
- ☐ 20 sec: Low Push Up Pulse
- ☐ 10 sec: Rest

4th Set: 3 Rounds
- ☐ 20 sec: Slow Squat Jumps
- ☐ 10 sec: Rest
- ☐ 20 sec: Fast Squat Jumps
- ☐ 10 sec: Rest
- ☐ 20 sec: Low Plank
- ☐ 10 sec: Rest
- ☐ 20 sec: Low Plank with Alternating Leg Lift
- ☐ 10 sec: Rest

Workout #62

1st Set: 1 Round (Warm Up)
- [ ] 45 sec: Runners Lunge (R)
- [ ] 45 sec: Runners Lunge (L)

2nd Set: 2 Rounds
- [ ] 50 sec: Switch Kick Abs
- [ ] 10 sec: Rest
- [ ] 50 sec: Overhead Sit Ups
- [ ] 10 sec: Rest
- [ ] 50 sec: Jack Squats
- [ ] 10 sec: Rest

3rd Set: 3 Rounds
- [ ] 30 sec: Tricep Dip Reach
- [ ] 15 sec: One Legged Tricep Dip Reach (R)
- [ ] 15 sec: One Legged Tricep Dip Reach (L)
- [ ] 30 sec: Fast Bench Dips

4th Set: 3 Rounds
- [ ] 50 sec: 2 Lunges + 1 Squat
- [ ] 10 sec: Rest
- [ ] 50 sec: Push Up Rows
- [ ] 10 sec: Rest
- [ ] 50 sec: Star Jumps
- [ ] 10 sec: Rest
- [ ] 50 sec: Shoelace Crunches
- [ ] 10 sec: Rest

Workout #63

68

1st Set: 1 Round (Warm Up)
- ☐ 60 sec: Downward Dog
- ☐ 45 sec: Pigeon Pose (R)
- ☐ 45 sec: Pigeon Pose (L)

2nd Set: 3 Rounds
- ☐ 45 sec: Standing Switch Kicks
- ☐ 15 sec: Rest
- ☐ 45 sec: Lying Windshield Wipers
- ☐ 15 sec: Rest
- ☐ 45 sec: Glute Bridges
- ☐ 15 sec: Rest

3rd Set: 5 Rounds
- ☐ 15 Chair Pose Squats
- ☐ 15 Pike Push Ups
- ☐ 15 Bear Hug Crunches
- ☐ 10 Twisting Squat Jumps
- ☐ 10 Spiderman Push Ups
- ☐ 50 Calf Raises

Workout #64

1st Set: 1 Round (Warm Up)
- ☐ 60 sec: Down Dog Walk Outs
- ☐ 30 sec: Plank with Hip Twists

2nd Set: 5 Rounds
- ☐ 10 Push Ups
- ☐ 60 sec: Low Plank
- ☐ 10 Staggered Push Ups
- ☐ 30 sec: Side Plank (R)
- ☐ 10 Pike Push Ups
- ☐ 30 sec: Side Plank (L)

3rd Set: 5 Rounds
- ☐ 10 Jump Squats
- ☐ 60 sec: Overhead Reverse Lunges
- ☐ 10 Jump Squats
- ☐ 60 sec: Lying Leg Raises
- ☐ 10 Jump Squats
- ☐ 60 sec: Wall Sit with Alternating Heel Lift

Workout #65

1st Set: 1 Round (Warm Up)
- ☐ 45 sec: Glute Bridges
- ☐ 45 sec: Lunges with Upper Rotations

2nd Set: 3 Rounds
- ☐ 60 sec: Jump Rope
- ☐ 45 sec: Speed Skaters
- ☐ 15 sec: Rest
- ☐ 45 sec: Star Jumps
- ☐ 15 sec: Rest
- ☐ 45 sec: Squat with Alternating Forward Kicks
- ☐ 15 sec: Rest
- ☐ 45 sec: Mountain Climbers
- ☐ 15 sec: Rest
- ☐ 45 sec: High Knee Run
- ☐ 15 sec: Rest
- ☐ 45 sec: Bench Jump Overs
- ☐ 15 sec: Rest
- ☐ 45 sec: Slow Push Ups
- ☐ 15 sec: Rest

3rd Set: 3 Rounds
- ☐ 30 sec: Wall Sit
- ☐ 30 sec: Low Plank
- ☐ 30 sec: Glute Bridge Hold
- ☐ 30 sec: Superman Hold

Workout #66

1st Set: 1 Round (Warm Up)
- ☐ 60 sec: Arm Circles
- ☐ 60 sec: Side-to-Side Lunge Stretch

2nd Set: 3 Rounds
- ☐ 30 Wide Push Ups from Knees
- ☐ 30 Squats
- ☐ 30 sec: Side Plank (R)
- ☐ 30 sec: Side Plank (L)

3rd Set: 3 Rounds
- ☐ 60 sec: High Knee Run
- ☐ 60 sec: In-n-Out Squats
- ☐ 30 sec: Burpees
- ☐ 30 sec: Rest

4th Set: 1 Round
- ☐ Push Ups Until Failure
- ☐ Air Squats Until Failure

Workout #67

1st Set: 2 Rounds (Warm Up)
- ☐ 10 Hip Openers (R)
- ☐ 10 Hip Openers (L)
- ☐ 10 Frankenstein Kicks (R)
- ☐ 10 Frankenstein Kicks (L)

2nd Set: 3 Rounds
- ☐ 30 sec: Low Plank
- ☐ 30 sec: Low Plank Jacks
- ☐ 30 sec: High Plank
- ☐ 30 sec: High Plank Jacks
- ☐ 30 sec: Slow Push Ups
- ☐ 30 sec: Push Up Jacks
- ☐ 30 sec: Low Push Up Pulses
- ☐ 30 sec: Rest
- ☐ 30 sec: Squats
- ☐ 30 sec: Low Squat Hold
- ☐ 30 sec: Low Squat Pulses
- ☐ 30 sec: Single Leg Lunges (R)
- ☐ 30 sec: Single Leg Lunge Hold (R)
- ☐ 30 sec: Single Leg Lunges (L)
- ☐ 30 sec: Single Leg Lunge Hold (L)
- ☐ 30 sec: Rest

3rd Set: 2 Rounds
- ☐ Burpees Until Failure
- ☐ 60 sec: Rest

Workout #68

1st Set: 2 Round (Warm Up)
- [ ] 30 sec: Standing Knee Hugs
- [ ] 30 sec: Butt Kicks
- [ ] 60 sec: Plank

2nd Set: 2 Rounds
- [ ] 50 sec: Forward Lunges
- [ ] 10 sec: Rest
- [ ] 50 sec: Lateral Lunges
- [ ] 10 sec: Rest
- [ ] 50 sec: Reverse Lunges
- [ ] 10 sec: Rest
- [ ] 50 sec: Curtsey Lunges
- [ ] 10 sec: Rest

3rd Set: 2 Rounds
- [ ] 50 sec: High Plank
- [ ] 10 sec: Rest
- [ ] 50 sec: Low Plank
- [ ] 10 sec: Rest
- [ ] 50 sec: Wide Push Ups from Knees
- [ ] 10 sec: Rest
- [ ] 50 sec: Diamond Push Ups from Knees
- [ ] 10 sec: Rest

4th Set: 3 Rounds
- [ ] 30 sec: Shoelace Crunches
- [ ] 30 sec: Lying Leg Lifts
- [ ] 30 sec: In-n-Out Abs
- [ ] 30 sec: Russian Twists
- [ ] 30 sec: Boat Pose Hold

Workout #69

74

1st Set: 1 Round (Warm Up)
- ☐ 60 sec: Downward Dog
- ☐ 30 sec: Runners Stretch (R)
- ☐ 30 sec: Runners Stretch (L)

2nd Set: 1 Round
- ☐ 100 Mountain Climbers (50 each side)
- ☐ 90 High Knee Run (45 each side)
- ☐ 80 Crunches
- ☐ 70 Air Squats
- ☐ 60 Alternating Reverse Lunges (30 each side)
- ☐ 50 Seal Jacks
- ☐ 40 Push Ups
- ☐ 30 Plank Jacks
- ☐ 20: Jump Squats
- ☐ 10: Burpees

Workout #70

75

1st Set: 3 Rounds (Warm Up)
- [ ] 12 Air Squats
- [ ] 12 Push Ups
- [ ] 12 Mountain Climbers

2nd Set: 3 Rounds
- [ ] 30 Plank Side Punches (15 each side)
- [ ] 30 sec: Plank Shoulder Taps
- [ ] 20 Jumping Lunges (10 each side)
- [ ] 20 sec: Standing Side Kicks
- [ ] 10 Wide Push Ups
- [ ] 10 sec: Low Pulsing Push Ups

3rd Set: 3 Rounds
- [ ] 30 sec: Up and Down Planks
- [ ] 30 sec: Squat + Alternating Side Kick
- [ ] 30 sec: Scissor Kicks
- [ ] 30 sec: Fire Hydrants (R)
- [ ] 30 sec: Fire Hydrants (L)
- [ ] 30 sec: Lying Leg Windshield Wipers
- [ ] 30 sec: Rest

Workout #71

1st Set: 2 Rounds (Warm Up)
- ☐ 30 sec: Chest Expansions
- ☐ 30 sec: Standing Half Jacks
- ☐ 30 sec: Torso Rotations

2nd Set: 1 Round
- ☐ 20 Squat + 2 Punches
- ☐ 10 Plank Toe Taps
- ☐ 20 Squat + 2 Punches
- ☐ 10 Supermans
- ☐ 20 Squat + 2 Punches
- ☐ 10 Diamond Push Ups
- ☐ 20 Squat + 2 Punches
- ☐ 10 Seal Jacks
- ☐ 20 Squat + 2 Punches
- ☐ 10 Roller Coasters
- ☐ 20 Squat + 2 Punches
- ☐ 10 Plank Walk Outs

3rd Set: 1 Round
- ☐ 20 Plank Shoulder Taps (10 each side)
- ☐ 10 Butterfly Crunches
- ☐ 20 Plank Shoulder Taps
- ☐ 10 V-Ups
- ☐ 20 Plank Shoulder Taps
- ☐ 10 Single Leg Lunge (R)
- ☐ 20 Plank Shoulder Taps
- ☐ 10 Single Leg Lunge (L)
- ☐ 20 Plank Shoulder Taps
- ☐ 10 Lying Leg Lifts
- ☐ 20 Plank Shoulder Taps
- ☐ 10 Burpees

Workout #72

1st Set: 2 Rounds (Warm Up)
- ☐ 30 sec: High Knee Run
- ☐ 60 sec: Pigeon Pose (R)
- ☐ 60 sec: Pigeon Pose (R)

2nd Set: 3 Rounds
- ☐ 60 sec: Squats
- ☐ 30 sec: Staggered Push Ups
- ☐ 30 sec: Supermans
- ☐ 30 sec: Burpees
- ☐ 30 sec: Rest

3rd Set: 4 Rounds
- ☐ 8 Push Ups
- ☐ 8 L-Sit Ups
- ☐ 8 Single Leg Deadlift (L)
- ☐ 8 Single Leg Deadlift (R)
- ☐ 8 Tuck Jumps
- ☐ 8 Slow Mountain Climbers
- ☐ 30 sec: Rest

Workout #73

1st Set: 2 Rounds (Warm Up)
- ☐ 10 Neck Rotations
- ☐ 10 Torso Rotations
- ☐ 10 Single Leg Hip Rotation (R)
- ☐ 10 Single Leg Hip Rotation (L)

2nd Set: 1 Round
- ☐ 100 Squats
- ☐ 80 Forward Lunges (40 each side)
- ☐ 60 Heel Tap Crunches (30 each side)
- ☐ 40 Wide Push Ups
- ☐ 20 Burpees
- ☐ 40 Diamond Push Ups
- ☐ 60 Russian Twists (30 each side)
- ☐ 80 Reverse Lunges (40 each side)
- ☐ 100 Sumo Squats

Workout #74

1st Set: 2 Rounds (Warm Up)
- ☐ 30 sec: Standing Mountain Climbers
- ☐ 30 sec: Inch Worms
- ☐ 60 sec: Standing Alternating Toe Taps

2nd Set: 3 Rounds
- ☐ 45 sec: Overhead Squats
- ☐ 15 sec: Rest
- ☐ 45 sec: Sumo Squat Low Hold
- ☐ 15 sec: Rest
- ☐ 45 sec: 4 High Knees + 4 Punches
- ☐ 15 sec: Rest
- ☐ 30 sec: Reverse Lunges with Knee Drive (R)
- ☐ 30 sec: Reverse Lunges with Knee Drive (L)

3rd Set: 3 Rounds
- ☐ 45 sec: Back and Forth Planks
- ☐ 15 sec: Rest
- ☐ 45 sec: Flutter Kicks
- ☐ 15 sec: Rest
- ☐ 45 sec: Spiderman Push Ups
- ☐ 15 sec: Rest
- ☐ 30 sec: Side Plank with Hip Dips (R)
- ☐ 30 sec: Side Plank with Hip Dips (L)

Workout #75

1st Set: 2 Rounds (Warm Up)
- ☐ 30 sec: Bird Dogs
- ☐ 30 sec: Cat Cow Pose
- ☐ 60 sec: Jump Rope

2nd Set: 5 Rounds
- ☐ 15 Burpees
- ☐ 10 Single Leg Lunge (R)
- ☐ 10 Single Leg Lunge (L)
- ☐ 15 Low Squat Jacks
- ☐ 10 Slow Push Ups
- ☐ 15 Shoelace Crunches
- ☐ 10 Plank Jacks
- ☐ 15 Tuck Jumps
- ☐ 10 Supermans

Workout #76

1st Set: 1 Round (Warm Up)
- ☐ 30 sec: Small Arm Circles
- ☐ 30 sec: Hip Circles
- ☐ 30 sec: Big Arm Circles
- ☐ 30 sec: Frankenstein Kicks

2nd Set: 2 Rounds
- ☐ 50 Reverse Lunge Knee Taps (25 each side)
- ☐ 40 Cross Body Mountain Climbers
- ☐ 30 Ski Hops
- ☐ 20 Burpees
- ☐ Plyo Push Ups

3rd Set: 3 Rounds
- ☐ 50 sec: One Legged Deadlifts (R)
- ☐ 10 sec: Rest
- ☐ 50 sec: One Legged Deadlifts (L)
- ☐ 10 sec: Rest
- ☐ 30 sec: Slow Push Ups
- ☐ 30 sec: Low Plank with Hip Twist

82

1st Set: 2 Rounds (Warm Up)
- ☐ 60 sec: Jump Rope
- ☐ 60 sec: Incline Push Ups

2nd Set: 3 Rounds
- ☐ 45 sec: Cocoons
- ☐ 15 sec: Low Plank
- ☐ 45 sec: Wall Sit with Heels Lifts
- ☐ 15 sec: Low Plank
- ☐ 45 sec: Cross Body Crunches
- ☐ 15 sec: Low Plank
- ☐ 45 sec: Bench Dips
- ☐ 15 sec: Low Plank

3rd Set: 5 Rounds
- ☐ 20 sec: Reverse Crunches
- ☐ 10 sec: High Plank
- ☐ 20 sec: Glute Bridge Hold
- ☐ 10 sec: High Plank
- ☐ 20 sec: Burpees
- ☐ 10 sec: High Plank
- ☐ 20 sec: Jump Squats
- ☐ 10 sec: High Plank

Workout #78

1st Set: 1 Round (Warm Up)
- ☐ 50 Side to Side Hops
- ☐ 40 High Knees (20 each side)
- ☐ 30 Russian Twists (15 each side)
- ☐ 20 Squats
- ☐ 10 Push Ups

2nd Set: 3 Rounds
- ☐ 20: 5-Way Push Ups
- ☐ 20: Ab Choppers (10 each side)
- ☐ 20: Alternating Fire Hydrants (10 each side)
- ☐ 20: Alternating Side Planks (10 each side)
- ☐ 20: Squat to Basketball Shots (10 each side)

3rd Set: 3 Rounds
- ☐ 30 sec: Butt Kicks
- ☐ 30 sec: Jumping Jacks
- ☐ 30 sec: In-n-Out Squats
- ☐ 30 sec: Frog Burpees
- ☐ 30 sec: Pike Push Ups
- ☐ 30 sec: Rest

Workout #79

1st Set: 1 Round (Warm Up)
- ☐ 25 Jumping Jacks
- ☐ 25 Squats
- ☐ 25 Push Ups
- ☐ 25 Crunches

2nd Set: 5 Rounds
- ☐ 5 Jump Squats
- ☐ 10 Butterfly Crunches
- ☐ 15 Wide Push Ups
- ☐ 10 Lying Leg Lifts
- ☐ 5 Burpee Tuck Jumps
- ☐ 30 sec: Rest

3rd Set: 3 Rounds
- ☐ 50 sec: Crunchy Frogs
- ☐ 10 sec: Jumping Jacks
- ☐ 50 sec: Curtsy Lunges
- ☐ 10 sec: Frog Burpees
- ☐ 50 sec: Diamond Push Ups from Knees
- ☐ 10 sec: Rest

Workout #80

1st Set: 1 Round (Warm Up)
- ☐ 30 sec: High Plank
- ☐ 30 sec: Side Plank (R)
- ☐ 30 sec: Low Plank
- ☐ 30 sec: Side Plank (L)

2nd Set: 1 Round
- ☐ 100 Squats
- ☐ 80 Calf Raises
- ☐ 60 Push Ups
- ☐ 40 Plank Shoulder Taps (20 each side)
- ☐ 20 Lying Scissor Kicks (10 each side)

3rd Set: 3 Rounds
- ☐ 20 sec: Supermans
- ☐ 10 sec: Rest
- ☐ 20 sec: Elbow to Knee Bird Dogs (R)
- ☐ 10 sec: Rest
- ☐ 20 sec: Elbow to Knee Bird Dogs (L)
- ☐ 10 sec: Rest

Workout #81

1st Set: 1 Round (Warm Up)
- ☐ 10 Slow Push Ups
- ☐ 10 Slow Squats
- ☐ 10 Slow Crunches

2nd Set: 2 Rounds
- ☐ 20 Wide Push Ups
- ☐ 20 Sumo Squats
- ☐ 20 Shoelace Crunches

3rd Set: 2 Rounds
- ☐ 20 Diamond Push Ups
- ☐ 20 Close Squats
- ☐ 20 Knees Up Crunches

4th Set: 3 Rounds
- ☐ 30 Fast Push Ups
- ☐ 30 Fast Squats
- ☐ 30 Russian Twists (15 each side)

Workout #82

1st Set: 1 Round (Warm Up)
- ☐ 60 sec: Inch Worms
- ☐ 60 sec: Downward Dog

2nd Set: 2 Rounds
- ☐ 50 sec: High Plank Jacks
- ☐ 10 sec: Rest
- ☐ 50 sec: Glute Bridges
- ☐ 10 sec: Rest
- ☐ 50 sec: Froggy Jumps
- ☐ 10 sec: Rest

3rd Set: 3 Rounds
- ☐ 45 sec: Low Plank with Alternating Leg Lifts
- ☐ 15 sec: Rest
- ☐ 45 sec: Glute Reverse Lunges
- ☐ 15 sec: Rest
- ☐ 45 sec: Squat with Alternating Front Kick
- ☐ 15 sec: Rest

4th Set: 3 Rounds
- ☐ 20 sec: Fast Mountain Climbers
- ☐ 10 sec: Rest
- ☐ 20 sec: Jumping Lunges
- ☐ 10 sec: Rest
- ☐ 20 sec: Push Up + 2 Shoulder Taps
- ☐ 10 sec: Rest

Workout #83

1st Set: 1 Round (Warm Up)
- ☐ 30 sec: Forward Lunges
- ☐ 30 sec: Reverse Lunges
- ☐ 30 sec: Lateral Lunges
- ☐ 60 sec: Downward Dog Push Ups

2nd Set: 2 Rounds
- ☐ 90 sec: Jump Rope
- ☐ 30 sec: L-Seat Lift
- ☐ 60 sec: Standing Side-to-Side Kicks
- ☐ 90 sec: Wall Sit
- ☐ 30 sec: High Plank Alternating Front Raise
- ☐ 60 sec: Burpee Jump Overs

3rd Set: 5 Rounds
- ☐ 20 sec: Lying One Legged Hold (R)
- ☐ 10 sec: Rest
- ☐ 20 sec: Lying One Legged Hold (L)
- ☐ 10 sec: Rest
- ☐ 20 sec: Side Plank with Hip Dips (R)
- ☐ 10 sec: Rest
- ☐ 20 sec: Side Plank with Hip Dips (L)
- ☐ 10 sec: Rest

Workout #84

1st Set: 1 Round (Warm Up)
- ☐ 45 sec: Side to Side Leg Swings (R)
- ☐ 45 sec: Side to Side Leg Swings (L)
- ☐ 45 sec: Downward Dog
- ☐ 45 sec: Child's Pose

2nd Set: 3 Rounds
- ☐ 20: Front to Back One Legged Lunge (R)
- ☐ 20: Front to Back One Legged Lunge (R)
- ☐ 15: One Legged Mountain Climber (R)
- ☐ 15: One Legged Mountain Climber (L)
- ☐ 10: Decline Push Ups
- ☐ 10: Incline Push Ups
- ☐ 30 sec: Rest

3rd Set: 3 Rounds
- ☐ 50 sec: Reverse Plank
- ☐ 10 sec: Rest
- ☐ 50 sec: Speed Skaters
- ☐ 10 sec: Rest
- ☐ 50 sec: 2 Lunges + 1 Squat
- ☐ 10 sec: Rest
- ☐ 50 sec: Push Up + 2 Shoulder Taps
- ☐ 10 sec: Rest

Workout #85

1st Set: 1 Round (Warm Up)
- ☐ 30 sec: Jump Rope
- ☐ 30 sec: Jumping Jacks
- ☐ 30 sec: Forward Lunges with Twist
- ☐ 30 sec: Russian Twists

2nd Set: 3 Rounds
- ☐ 60 sec: Sumo Squats
- ☐ 20 Jump Squats
- ☐ 60 sec: Low Plank Jacks
- ☐ 20 Fast Push Ups
- ☐ 60 sec: High Plank with Alternating Row
- ☐ 20 Supermans
- ☐ 60 sec: Hollow Body Hold
- ☐ 20 Shoelace Crunches

3rd Set: 1 Round
- ☐ 60 sec: Burpees
- ☐ 60 sec: Low Plank

Workout #86

1st Set: 1 Round (Warm Up)
- ☐ 30 High Knees (15 each side)
- ☐ 30 Butt Kicks (15 each side)
- ☐ 30 Jumping Jacks
- ☐ 10 Push Ups

2nd Set: 10 Rounds
- ☐ 10 Long Crunches
- ☐ 10 Jumping Lunges (5 each side)
- ☐ 10 Lying Leg Figure 8's
- ☐ 10 Supermans
- ☐ 10 Slow Push Ups

3rd Set: 2 Rounds
- ☐ 30 sec: Mummy Kicks
- ☐ 30 sec: Plyo Jacks
- ☐ 30 sec: Pike Push Ups
- ☐ 30 sec: Plank Lateral Walk
- ☐ 30 sec: Rest

Workout #87

1st Set: 1 Round (Warm Up)
- ☐ 60 sec: Prisoner Squats
- ☐ 45 sec: High Side Plank (R)
- ☐ 45 sec: High Side Plank (L)
- ☐ 30 sec: Bicycle Crunches

2nd Set: 3 Rounds
- ☐ 40 sec: Push Up Knee Tucks
- ☐ 20 sec: Rest
- ☐ 40 sec: Squat Jumps (Slow going down, Explosive going up)
- ☐ 20 sec: Rest
- ☐ 40 sec: Alternating Low Side Plank
- ☐ 20 sec: Rest
- ☐ 40 sec: Lying Rotating Leg Lifts
- ☐ 20 sec: Rest
- ☐ 40 sec: High Knee Sprint
- ☐ 20 sec: Rest

3rd Set: 1 Rounds
- ☐ 50 Squats
- ☐ 50 Push Ups
- ☐ 50 sec: Plank

Workout #88

1st Set: 1 Round (Warm Up)
- ☐ 60 sec: Downward Dog
- ☐ 60 sec: Glute Bridge Hold
- ☐ 30 sec: Pigeon Pose (R)
- ☐ 30 sec: Pigeon Pose (R)

2nd Set: 5 Rounds
- ☐ 10 Frog Burpees
- ☐ 9 Jump Squats
- ☐ 8 Wide Push Ups
- ☐ 7 Seal Jacks
- ☐ 6 Lying Leg Lifts
- ☐ 5 Diamond Push Ups
- ☐ 4 Mountain Climbers (4 each side)
- ☐ 3 Tuck Jumps
- ☐ 2 Squats
- ☐ 1 min: Jump Rope

Workout #89

1st Set: 1 Round (Warm Up)
- ☐ 60 sec: Jumping Jacks
- ☐ 60 sec: Mountain Climbers
- ☐ 30 sec: Straight Leg Stretch (R)
- ☐ 30 sec: Straight Leg Stretch (L)

2nd Set: 1 Round
- ☐ 30 Cross Punch Crunches (15 each side)
- ☐ 21 Jump Tucks
- ☐ 21 Low Pulsing Push Ups
- ☐ 30 Bicycle Crunches (15 each side)
- ☐ 18 Bench Jump Overs
- ☐ 18 Push Ups from Knees
- ☐ 30 Crunchy Frogs
- ☐ 15 Froggy Jumps
- ☐ 15 Incline Push Ups
- ☐ 30 Reverse Crunches
- ☐ 12 Star Jumps
- ☐ 12 Decline Push Ups
- ☐ 30 Overhead Crunches
- ☐ 9 Sumo Squat Jumps
- ☐ 9 Plyo Push Ups
- ☐ 30 Diamond Crunches
- ☐ 6 Jumping Lunges
- ☐ 6 Spiderman Push Ups
- ☐ 30 In-n-Out Crunches
- ☐ 3 Burpee Tuck Jumps
- ☐ 3 Slow Push Ups

Workout #90

1st Set: 3 Rounds (Warm Up)
- ☐ 10 Lunges
- ☐ 10 Squats
- ☐ 10 Wide Push Ups

2nd Set: 3 Rounds
- ☐ 60 sec: Jump Rope
- ☐ 20 Prisoner Squats
- ☐ 20 Lying Scissor Kicks (10 each side)
- ☐ 30 sec: Rest

3rd Set: 3 Rounds
- ☐ 45 sec: Burpees
- ☐ 15 Slow Push Ups
- ☐ 15 Mountain Climbers
- ☐ 30 sec: Rest

3rd Set: 3 Rounds
- ☐ 30 sec: Jump Squats
- ☐ 10 One Legged Lying Leg Lifts (R)
- ☐ 10 One Legged Lying Leg Lifts (L)
- ☐ 30 sec: Rest

Workout #91

1st Set: 1 Round (Warm Up)
- ☐ 60 sec: Inchworms
- ☐ 30 sec: Standing Toe Taps
- ☐ 30 sec: Plank Toe Taps

2nd Set: 3 Rounds
- ☐ 45 sec: High Knee Jog
- ☐ 15 sec: High Plank
- ☐ 45 sec: Elevator Squats
- ☐ 15 sec: High Plank
- ☐ 45 sec: 1 Squat + 4 Reverse Lunges
- ☐ 15 sec: High Plank
- ☐ 45 sec: Ski Hops
- ☐ 15 sec: High Plank
- ☐ 45 sec: Low Squat Pulses
- ☐ 15 sec: High Plank

3rd Set: 3 Rounds
- ☐ 40 sec: Modified Burpees
- ☐ 20 sec: Wall Sit
- ☐ 40 sec: Push Ups from Knees
- ☐ 20 sec: Wall Sit
- ☐ 40 sec: Bench Dips
- ☐ 20 sec: Wall Sit
- ☐ 40 sec: Pike Push Ups
- ☐ 20 sec: Wall Sit
- ☐ 40 sec: Supermans
- ☐ 20 sec: Wall Sit

Workout #92

1st Set: 1 Round (Warm Up)
- ☐ 20 Jumping Jacks
- ☐ 16 Forward Lunges with Twist
- ☐ 12 Squat to Overhead Reach
- ☐ 8 Downward Dog Push Ups

2nd Set: 3 Rounds
- ☐ 30 sec: Deep Squats
- ☐ 30 sec: Slow Mountain Climbers
- ☐ 30 sec: Glute Kickbacks (R)
- ☐ 30 sec: Glute Kickbacks (L)
- ☐ 30 sec: Low Plank with Alternating Leg Lifts
- ☐ 30 sec: Rest

3rd Set: 3 Rounds
- ☐ 30 sec: Plank to Push Ups
- ☐ 30 sec: Heel Tap Crunches
- ☐ 30 sec: One Legged Vertical Crunch (R)
- ☐ 30 sec: One Legged Vertical Crunch (L)
- ☐ 30 sec: Oblique Crunches (R)
- ☐ 30 sec: Oblique Crunches (L)

Workout #93

1st Set: 1 Round (Warm Up)
- ☐ 60 sec: Cat Cows
- ☐ 60 sec: Runners Lunge

2nd Set: 2 Rounds
- ☐ 50 sec: Fast Jumping Jacks
- ☐ 10 sec: Rest
- ☐ 50 sec: Wall Sit with Alternating Heel Lift
- ☐ 10 sec: Rest
- ☐ 50 sec: Fast Push Ups from Knees
- ☐ 10 sec: Rest
- ☐ 50 sec: Knees Up Crunches
- ☐ 10 sec: Rest
- ☐ 50 sec: Bench Step Ups
- ☐ 10 sec: Rest
- ☐ 50 sec: Bench Dips
- ☐ 10 sec: Rest
- ☐ 50 sec: Low Plank with Alternating Knee Taps
- ☐ 10 sec: Rest

3rd Set: 5 Rounds
- ☐ 20 sec: Full Push Ups
- ☐ 10 sec: Rest
- ☐ 20 sec: Deep Squats
- ☐ 10 sec: Rest

Workout #93

1st Set: 1 Round (Warm Up)
- [ ] 30 sec: Arm Circles
- [ ] 30 sec: Torso Rotations
- [ ] 30 sec: Hip Openers
- [ ] 30 sec: Front-to-Back Leg Swings (R)
- [ ] 30 sec: Front-to-Back Leg Swings (L)
- [ ] 30 sec: Shoulder Rolls

2nd Set: 3 Rounds
- [ ] 25 Prisoner Squats
- [ ] 25 Overhead Sit Ups
- [ ] 20 Curtsy Lunges (10 each side)
- [ ] 20 Shoelace Crunches
- [ ] 30 sec: Rest

3rd Set: 3 Rounds
- [ ] 30 sec: Flutter Kicks
- [ ] 30 sec: Lying Floor Wipers
- [ ] 30 sec: Lying Straight Leg Hip Raises
- [ ] 30 sec: Low Plank
- [ ] 30 sec: Push Ups
- [ ] 30 sec: Cross Body Mountain Climbers
- [ ] 30 sec: Bird Dogs
- [ ] 30 sec: Rest

Workout #94

1st Set: 1 Round (Warm Up)
- [ ] 45 sec: High Knee Jog
- [ ] 45 sec: Butt Kicks
- [ ] 45 sec: Cat Cows
- [ ] 45 sec: Downward Dog

2nd Set: 3 Rounds
- [ ] 50 sec: Low Plank with Leg Lifts
- [ ] 10 sec: Rest
- [ ] 50 sec: Single Legged Glute Bridges (R)
- [ ] 10 sec: Rest
- [ ] 50 sec: Single Legged Glute Bridges (L)
- [ ] 10 sec: Rest
- [ ] 50 sec: Sumo Squats
- [ ] 10 sec: Rest

3rd Set: 1 Round
- [ ] 10 Diamond Push Ups
- [ ] 20 Side Plank Hip Dips (R)
- [ ] 20 Side Plank Hip Dips (L)
- [ ] 30 High Plank Jacks
- [ ] 40 Bicycle Crunches (20 each side)
- [ ] 50 Burpees

Workout #95

1st Set: 1 Round (Warm Up)
- ☐ 60 sec: Standing Lateral Leg Lifts
- ☐ 60 sec: Slow Push Ups

2nd Set: 3 Rounds
- ☐ 40 Glute Kickbacks (20 each side)
- ☐ 40 Squat Pulses
- ☐ 40 Plank Shoulder Taps (20 each side)
- ☐ 40 Glute Bridges
- ☐ 40 Jumping Lunges (20 each side)
- ☐ 60 sec: Rest

3rd Set: 3 Round
- ☐ 20 sec: Chair Pose Jumps
- ☐ 10 sec: Rest
- ☐ 20 sec: Straight Legged Crunches
- ☐ 10 sec: Rest
- ☐ 20 sec: Rotating Low Plank
- ☐ 10 sec: Rest
- ☐ 20 sec: Squat with Oblique Crunch (R)
- ☐ 10 sec: Rest
- ☐ 20 sec: Squat with Oblique Crunch (L)
- ☐ 10 sec: Rest

Workout #96

1st Set: 1 Round (Warm Up)
- ☐ 30 sec: Straight Arm Side Bends
- ☐ 30 sec: Standing Knee Pulls
- ☐ 30 sec: Reverse Lunges
- ☐ 30 sec: Bird Dogs

2nd Set: 2 Rounds
- ☐ 40 sec: Fast Push Ups
- ☐ 20 sec: Rest
- ☐ 40 sec: Back-and-Forth Low Plank
- ☐ 20 sec: Rest
- ☐ 40 sec: High Plank with Front Raises
- ☐ 20 sec: Rest
- ☐ 40 sec: Dolphin Push Ups
- ☐ 20 sec: Rest
- ☐ 40 sec: Tricep Dips
- ☐ 20 sec: Rest

3rd Set: 2 Rounds
- ☐ 40 sec: One Legged Jumping Lunges (R)
- ☐ 20 sec: Rest
- ☐ 40 sec: One Legged Jumping Lunges (L)
- ☐ 20 sec: Rest
- ☐ 40 sec: Lying Straight Leg Pulses
- ☐ 20 sec: Rest
- ☐ 40 sec: Lying Scissor Kicks
- ☐ 20 sec: Rest
- ☐ 40 sec: Slow Squats
- ☐ 20 sec: Rest

Workout #97

1st Set: 1 Round (Warm Up)
- ☐ 60 sec: Hero Pose with Neck Rotations
- ☐ 60 sec: Yogi Squat
- ☐ 60 sec: Straight Leg Forward Fold

2nd Set: 2 Rounds
- ☐ 30 Froggy Jumps
- ☐ 30 Supermans
- ☐ 30 Star Jumps
- ☐ 30 Squats
- ☐ 30 Plank Toe Taps (15 each side)
- ☐ 30 Single Legged Deadlift (R)
- ☐ 30 Single Legged Deadlift (L)
- ☐ 30 Staggered Push Ups
- ☐ 30 Burpees

Workout #98

1st Set: 3 Rounds (Warm Up)
- ☐ 10 Push Ups
- ☐ 10 Sit Ups
- ☐ 10 Squats

2nd Set: 3 Rounds
- ☐ 40 sec: Jumping Lunges
- ☐ 20 sec: Rest
- ☐ 40 sec: Overhead Squats
- ☐ 20 sec: Rest
- ☐ 40 sec: Runners Lunges
- ☐ 20 sec: Rest
- ☐ 40 sec: Sumo Squats
- ☐ 20 sec: Rest
- ☐ 40 sec: Curtsy Lunges
- ☐ 20 sec: Rest

3rd Set: 1 Round
- ☐ 80 Jumping Jacks
- ☐ 70 Mummy Kicks (35 each side)
- ☐ 60 Crunches
- ☐ 50 Push Ups
- ☐ 40 Burpees
- ☐ 30 Glute Bridges
- ☐ 20 Lying Leg Lifts
- ☐ 10 Spiderman Push Ups

Workout #99

1st Set: 3 Rounds (Warm Up)
- ☐ 60 sec: Side Shuffles
- ☐ 60 sec: Mountain Climbers
- ☐ 30 sec: High Knee Run

2nd Set: 2 Rounds
- ☐ 20 Back-and-Forth Squat Hops
- ☐ 20 Squat Thrusts
- ☐ 20 Rollercoaster Push Ups
- ☐ 20 Tricep Dip Reach
- ☐ 20 Flutter Kicks

3rd Set: 3 Rounds
- ☐ 30 sec: Burpees
- ☐ 30 sec: Slow Squats
- ☐ 30 sec: Squat with Front Kick (R)
- ☐ 30 sec: Squat with Front Kick (L)
- ☐ 30 sec: Plyo Push Ups from Knees
- ☐ 30 sec: Diamond Crunches
- ☐ 30 sec: Rest

Workout #100

1st Set: 1 Round (Warm Up)
- ☐ 60 sec: Child's Pose
- ☐ 60 sec: Downward Dog
- ☐ 60 sec: Cat Cows

2nd Set: 1 Round
- ☐ 100 High Knees (50 each side)
- ☐ 90 Walking Lunges (45 each side)
- ☐ 80 Air Squats
- ☐ 70 Heel Tap Crunches
- ☐ 60 Push Ups
- ☐ 50 Frogger Jumps
- ☐ 40 Lateral Lunges
- ☐ 30 Plyo Push Ups
- ☐ 20 Squat Jumps
- ☐ 10 Burpee Tuck Jumps

Workout #101

1st Set: 3 Rounds (Warm Up)
- ☐ 60 sec: Downward Dog with Peddling Heels
- ☐ 30 sec: Pigeon Pose (R)
- ☐ 30 sec: Pigeon Pose (L)

2nd Set: 10 Rounds
- ☐ 10 Jumping Lunges (5 each side)
- ☐ 10 Push Ups
- ☐ 10 Fast Mountain Climbers
- ☐ 10 Glute Bridges
- ☐ 10 Push Ups with Alternating Leg Lift
- ☐ 10 Plank Jacks
- ☐ 10 Jump Squats
- ☐ 10 Sumo Squats
- ☐ 10 Burpees
- ☐ 30 sec: Rest